A Sister's Diary

by Jodi Scheinfeld

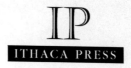

NEW YORK

Ithaca Press
3 Kimberly Drive, Suite B
Dryden, New York 13053 USA
www.IthacaPress.com

Cover Design	Gary Hoffman
Book Design	Gary Hoffman
Original art	Rachel Soboleski

Manufactured in the United States of America

9 8 7 6 5 4 3 2 1

Library of Congress Cataloging-in-Data Available
Scheinfeld/Jodi/ children/grief/death of a child/children's book about
grief

First Edition

Printed in the United States of America

ISBN 978-0-9825971-0-1

www.JodiScheinfeld.com

July 20
8:15 at night

Dear Diary,

Lots of people, including Aunt Mandy and Grandma Ruth, have given me blank books for writing and drawing over the past few weeks, but I've chosen you to be my silent friend. I like your cover the best of them all because yours is blank—pure white—until, of course, *I* decide to illustrate it with the gigantic set of colored pencils that you came with.

Does it seem like I'm not telling you what I really need to tell you? I hope you're patient because it will take me a long time to get all my feelings out.

I guess I should start with who I am and stuff like that, especially since I'm about to explain some things that are really private. Private. Private. Private. I'm Jessica Allman and I'm nine years old. I used to think a lot about my friends and my frog collection (stuffed animals, that is) and becoming a singer when I grow up. But my thoughts are really different these days. You see, something really terrible happened in my family and my old thoughts don't feel right anymore. My old thoughts belonged to the happy Jessica.

My dad is coming in my room to kiss me goodnight, so I'll have to save the rest of this story for tomorrow. I promise I'll tell you everything. Gee, I feel better already because I'm able to talk about stuff with you.

Your new friend,
Jessica

July 21

7:30 in the morning

Dear Diary,

At first I thought I would write to you only at the end of each day, but since I'm in the middle of a very important story, I thought I should get back to you right away. I didn't even go downstairs for breakfast yet, but what I'm about to tell you is much more important than eating.

You'll never be ready to hear this so I'll just come right out with it.

It's hard for me to come right out with it.

I never realized that putting things down on paper makes them even realer.

I wish this weren't real.

O.k.

Deep breath. My dad recommends deep breaths for tough times.

My older brother Matt passed away a few weeks ago. Do you know what "passed away" means? People around here say it that way, maybe because it sounds better than what it really means. It means . . . he died.

He was just about to turn eleven years old and he didn't always want to play with nine year-old me or anything. But he was my big brother who knew all the things I didn't know and he looked out for me during the important times and, Diary, he really died. He went to this overnight camp with horribly stupid counselors. They let him swim in the kind of water that pulls you under, sort of like the ocean does, but this was more like a wild river. He got pulled under and he couldn't breathe for a long time so his heart stopped beating and he couldn't be alive anymore. I really miss Matt and I feel really bad for him. I feel really bad for everyone around here. There's lots of crying all the time and different people take care of my other brothers and me most of the time, you know aunts, uncles, grandparents. My parents don't even feel like my parents because they just aren't with me very much now. This whole horrible story is making me feel like I don't want to write anymore today. I guess it's a good time to eat breakfast. I'm going to see if anyone else in the family is awake yet. Talk to you later. Hope you're not too upset.

Love ya,
Jessica

July 22

7:45 at night

Dear Diary,

You're probably wondering how I know exactly what time it is when I write to you. Well, the reason is sort of interesting so I'll tell you. My brother Matt had this really cool clock on his desk that our grandma gave him one year for his birthday. It had a radio and lots of colorful control buttons. Plus, it displayed the time of day in bright slime-green lights. He would play the radio each morning and dance around and sing while he got ready for school. If a good song came on, my brothers and I would hurry to his room and we'd all act like a band together, strumming imaginary guitars and blowing imaginary trumpets. We were kind of goofy but it was really fun.

Anyway, a few days ago when the house was feeling mouse quiet and I was missing the goofy times, I wandered into Matt's room and decided to sit at his desk for a little while. I've noticed that when I'm near his things I feel like he's right there with me. That probably sounds weird to you but it's true. Well, Diary, I barely breathed and I barely moved as I sat there like a paper clip on a magnet trying to feel his nearness. I wanted to open his drawers and touch whatever I might find in them, but I was sure my heart would stop beating altogether if I did that. So I only let myself look at the bright green light of his clock, and remember Matt singing along with its radio, soccer trophy in hand. He always grabbed this one trophy because its gleaming ball was just the right size for a microphone.

I decided I would ask my mom if I could keep Matt's clock next to my bed. I figured even if I didn't feel like playing music, I could look at the clock and be reminded of our band performances. So that's why I can always let you know what time it is, and you and I can both know that if it weren't for Matt, I wouldn't have a clock.

Hope you liked my Matt story. Maybe if I write lots of stories to you, you'll get to know him better. He was a great kid.

Signing off at 7:59.

Your friend,
Jessica

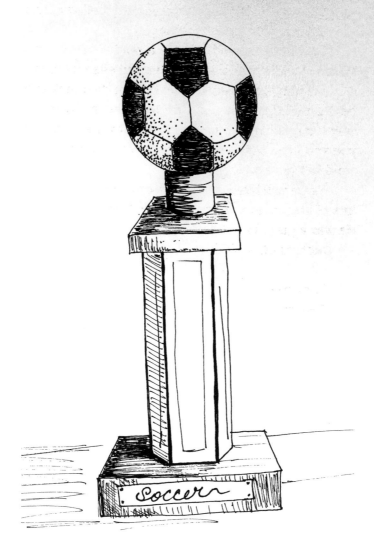

July 24
8:00 in the morning

Dear Diary,

Sorry I missed writing to you yesterday. We spent the day with Grandma Ruth and Grandpa Meyer and I was totally pooped at bedtime. I was thinking, though, that I haven't really told you about Ben and Ricky, my two other brothers who are missing Matt just as much as I am. Ben is seven years old with blue eyes and blond hair like me, except his hair is crew cut short and mine is middle of the back long. He actually shared a room with Matt, so I know this whole situation is pretty tough for him. He did a smart thing, though. He taped a picture on the wall exactly next to his pillow of Matt with Matt's best friend, Scott. Now Ben can remember Matt each night. Here is the super smart part: after he taped the picture next to his pillow, he took his camera and snapped a photo of the taped picture so he'd have an extra one for always. He told me and Ricky, "I'll make copies for you both so we can all have our own picture." That was nice of him. It's a really great picture with Matt and Scott wearing these tall Dr. Seuss hats and gigantic red tee- shirts. In case you're wondering, the hats and tee-shirts were costumes for their class play.

Ricky is our youngest but most talkative brother. He's not exactly a blabbermouth, but he does say exactly what's on his mind. He's four years old, has brown eyes and brown hair; honestly, he looks a lot like Matt when Matt was four. Ricky is all mixed up about what happened. He keeps asking if Matt will come back. The week after Matt passed away our family kept a memorial candle burning for seven days. Ricky said to my Dad, "Dad, I know what that candle is for. It's a wishing candle. We can all make a wish that Matt will come back." My Dad told Ricky that his idea was very loving but the candle could only help us remember Matt, not bring him back.

Ricky always has cool ideas.

Well, now you know a little about all my brothers. Lucky or unlucky I have no sisters to introduce to you so I'll sign off until tomorrow.

Friends always,
Jessica

July 25
7:38 at night

Dear Diary,

You're going to think I'm crazy but I keep thinking how it feels like Matt is still here, almost like he's just on vacation for a little while. This is the weirdest thing of all, Diary. His toothbrush is still in the bathroom. I've been noticing it there, and it makes my eyes all stingy. But I'm afraid to say anything to Mom and Dad about it. I've been trying not to upset them. When they cry, I feel even sadder and sort of scared, too. Maybe I should take care of this problem by myself—just slip the toothbrush in my pocket and hide it in Matt's desk or something.

On second thought, I'm pretty sure I'm not brave enough to take care of this situation alone. In fact, there's no way I'm slipping anything anywhere. No way! I have to let Matt's stuff be. Besides, it's not *so* bad looking at his toothbrush. Maybe it's easier to think of him as being on vacation for now. After I get used to that idea maybe I'll get used to the idea that he's really—gone from our world.

I can understand why Ricky keeps asking me and Ben freaky questions. "When will Matt come home? He has to come home by tomorrow, doesn't he?" I may be more grown up and understand things better than Ricky, but I have the feeling of Ricky's questions inside of me, too. I just know the real answer. Matt *won't* be coming home.

O.k. Diary. This is really mean of me. I can't let either of us go to sleep with such a sad thought. Here's a funny memory about Matt and me that my mom used to laugh about with us.

When I was a baby I was a really good eater, even though I'm a picky eater now. I would actually hum with each spoonful of sweet potatoes and green beans. "Hmm, hmm," like that. Even with mushy, squishy, yucky vegetables! One day I was eating spaghetti in my high chair, not too neatly but very happily. I must've had the reddish-orange sauce splattered all over my face. Matt was about three years old and he said to my mom, "Jessica looks like a carrot!" Nice compliment, huh?

Your favorite carrot face,
Jessica

July 26
5:25 before dinner

Dear Diary,

Would you like to know the best thing that happened today? I received a letter in the mail from my best friend, Lindsay Beth Silber. We've known each other since our diaper days when we were two years old. In nursery school we always played "house" with these two boys, Benny and Jeffie. Don't ask me why but our "house" had two bossy dads, Ben and Jeff, and two get-along great sisters, Lindsay and Jessica! Looking back on it, I guess there was no way either one of us would even *pretend* to marry Benny or Jeffie. A good decision based on the way those guys act nowadays! Even though Lindsay and I have never been in the same class since nursery school, we're still bff—best friends forever.

Anyway, Lindsay is visiting her grandparents in the country for the entire summer and boy do I miss her. We spent a few days together when her family came back from the country to be with us right after Matt passed away, but I wish she could've stayed with me forever. She really does feel like a sister sometimes, except I think we get along much better than sisters do! Unfortunately, she'll be visiting her grandparents for almost another whole month until school starts again. In one way, I hope the month zooms by, but then again it would be okay for it to pass turtle slow, too. You see I'm not sure I can go back to school after what happened to my family. Too many kids will be staring at me or asking me questions or who knows—they may be afraid to talk to me at all.

Well, I won't worry about that right now. Right now I'm going to enjoy my mail. Lindsay did promise to write me and she is one girl who always keeps a promise. Today's letter came in a bright pink envelope decorated with frog stickers, my favorite.

She wrote, "I *hope* you're not too sad about Matt but you *probably* are really sad." She's right, as usual! "I made this bracelet to cheer you up. Hope you like it."

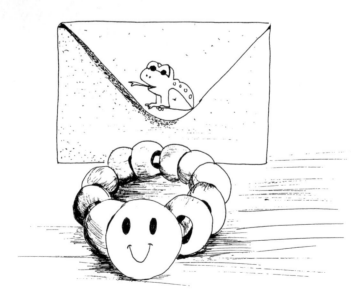

Of course I love it! It's made of golden yellow beads, except there's one smiley face bead in the middle. Actually, when I wear it I feel a little happy knowing I have a great friend who really cares about me. Lindsay is the only person I'd allow to read your pages, Diary.

I think I'll sign off for now and write her back.

Love,
Jessica

July 27
12:00, lunchtime

Dear Diary,

For some reason I spent much of the morning looking for places where I could write giant messages about Matt. I found these spots:

On my dresser mirror I wrote "Sorry Matt" in washable markers.

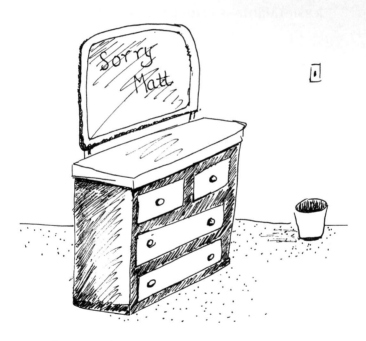

On my dry erase wall calendar across the month of July I wrote "I miss Mattie." (When he was smaller we called Matt "Mattie.")

On my chalkboard in the basement I wrote in the hugest letters of all "Matt, I wish you could come back. IT'S NOT FAIR!"

Since I erased all of these messages because I was afraid my parents would find them, I thought I should write a lasting message in you, Diary. That's all I feel like saying for today, except that it felt good to write those messages.

Thanks for being here,
Jessie (Mattie used to call me Jessie sometimes)

July 28
5:30 in the evening

Dear Diary,

Today this doctor lady named Faye came to our home to try to help our family feel better. That's a pretty impossible job! She told us we could just say what we were thinking to her and since she's worked with lots of families who have gone through sad things, she might be able to give a little advice.

Our whole family sat together with her on our screen porch. Ricky played with his cars through most of her visit and Ben kept asking for snacks, snacks and more snacks. I was getting kind of annoyed by what Ben and Ricky were doing. Our family felt like a mountain of broken glass and all Ben could do was ask for food, food, food. Ricky's only four so I could understand him playing with cars but Ben was really getting to me. They didn't seem to realize it was time to pay attention.

Anyway, I decided to speak up. "I have this bad feeling most of the time now, Faye, near where my heart beats. It's almost like I have frozen skin near my heart, not cold skin but stuck skin."

Ben and Ricky held still for a minute when I said this. Now they were listening. Faye seemed to understand what I meant and she made a really simple suggestion that I was glad she said in front of the whole family. Diary, according to Faye, "When you feel bad inside you should ask somebody close to you for a hug, a warm snug hug."

She was totally right. Nobody in our house had been hugging *at all* lately. We've been like ice cubes glued to the tray. I could've hugged Faye that very minute for her wonderful idea.

I'm going to ask Mom and Dad for a hug at bedtime tonight. I hope her idea really works.

Hugs to you, too.
Jessica

July 29

6:45 in the morning

Dear Diary,

It was really hot last night and I couldn't sleep so well. I just woke up and it's only 6:30 a.m. The whole house is still snoozing, so I thought I'd fill you in on a couple of things. At bedtime I did ask my mom and dad for big hugs. My dad hugged me so tight I had a little trouble breathing. But he's got this really great smell about him; I can't think of anything to compare it to but a warm, Dad, shaving cream-type smell, I guess. Mom gave me what she calls a "heartbeat to heartbeat" hug where we stay so close that we can feel the other person's heartbeat. That's a really great feeling. My mom always reminds me that when I was a baby she would hug me on the changing table and I wouldn't let her go, not if the phone rang, not if Matt started fussing, not even if she needed to pee. I guess I was born a hugger.

I'm feeling a little sad that I didn't give Mattie a hug too often. Maybe that's because boys don't do a lot of hugging—more smiling and joking and bouncing a ball, now that I think about it.

You know what I realized last night? I'm the oldest child in the family now. Doesn't that stink? It's like I'm the oldest one by age but I'll never be able to be the oldest like Mattie was. He knew how to handle things and give good advice about stuff.

He had no problem being the first Allman to board the school bus on opening day. Ben and I would always insist he get on first, kind of like a body guard, because we knew kids respected him, and they wouldn't dare try to tease us or trip us when we were rushing to find a seat. He would actually walk me and Ben to our classrooms for the first few days of school. It used to make me feel a little baby-ish, but I'm sure going to miss it this year. I wasn't supposed to be the oldest in the family. There's no way I can get on a bus without him walking in front of me. Maybe I can be homeschooled. Have you ever heard of that, Diary? I think a teacher comes to your house and you learn just as much as you would at school but without any kids to whisper about you.

I'm just going to go on as if I'm not the oldest. I'll have to let everyone in the family know how I feel about it, too. Well—not just yet. I might get Mom and Dad too sad. I'll talk to Ricky and Ben about it first. Speaking of whom, Ricky is now peeking in my doorway. He must've dressed himself last night because his pajamas are on backwards. He always wakes up with popping porcupine hair after sleeping. What a sight! Wish you could see it, too.

Love,
Jessica

July 30

7:23 at night

Dear Diary,

Right before dinner Ben, Ricky and I held our first kids' meeting since Matt passed away. You probably have no idea what I'm talking about so let me explain. We kids have had a tradition of meeting in Matt and Ben's room every once in a while to talk about stuff privately away from our parents' ears. Things like plans for Mom and Dad's birthdays, or ways to get along better if we've been fighting too much, or ideas for fun activities like the MJBR lemonade stand (M for Matt, J for Jessica, B for Ben and R for Ricky), that kind of stuff. Matt always led the meetings and I usually took notes. Ben sometimes offered good ideas but Ricky usually just hung out in the room, mostly playing and listening and saying silly things.

I've been missing our kids' meetings but I also felt really horrible about holding one without Matt. Today, though, I couldn't wait any longer, even if there was no leader for the meeting. I was desperate to let Ben and Ricky know that I refuse to be the oldest kid in our family. So we met after lunch in Matt and Ben's room and we sat in our usual places, but kind of glued to our seats. Diary, this might sound really strange but we also set up Matt's seat just as if he were part of it. We had to. We couldn't do it without him. It's very hard to explain how we felt.

Then I blurted it out. "I want you both to know that just because Matt's not here anymore, I refuse to be the oldest Allman kid. I don't know how to be it; I don't want to be it. So there!"

I think I shocked Ben and Ricky because they just stared at me speechless. Ricky looked a little confused and asked if he could still be the youngest. This made Ben and me laugh, and we assured him at the same time, "Of course you can, Ricky!" He looked very relieved, I felt much better and Ben, as usual, said he was hungry. Thankfully Mom called us downstairs for dinner at that very moment.

Between you and me, Diary, it was super hard to hold a kid's meeting without Matt. I hope it goes better next time. At least Ben and Ricky understand that I'm not and can never be the oldest Allman kid. Nope. Matt Allman will always be the oldest child in our family.

Love always,
Jessica

July 31

5:20 before dinner

Hi D,

Hope you don't mind if I use the initial "D" for you sometimes. I only use initials for friends I feel close to.

Can you smell anything? I guess not so I'll tell you what smells. I just took a shower and used a little bit of Matt's deodorant. It's not even like Matt wore deodorant all the time but he had gotten this sample of Old Spice at school during a workshop on growing up and taking care of your body. I know he used it before his elementary school graduation party in June. Ben and I smelled something funny on him that night but he wouldn't tell us what it was. Then I found the Old Spice on his desk after he'd left for the party and sure enough, that was the smell. I didn't even know what deodorant was until I had my mom explain this unidentified object to me.

I haven't told anyone in the family that I used Matt's Old Spice after my shower tonight. I simply stopped by Matt and Ben's room pretending to search for my hairbrush. I swiped the deodorant off Matt's desk, hurried into Matt's closet, rub-a-dub dubbed the spice right where they say you need it. Ever see a grownup with sweat stains by the armpits? That's where you need it. After checking that the coast was clear, I returned the bottle to the exact place I'd found it on Matt's desk.

For some reason, Diary, I don't mind fiddling with stuff *on* Matt's desk. Maybe it's because I'm used to seeing Matt's "on the desk" stuff. Looking inside his desk would be much harder, Diary. Even though it would bring me closer to him, I don't think my heart could handle it.

Anyway, I wonder if anyone will notice anything different about me tonight. Aunt Mandy is bringing over a macaroni and cheese dinner in a little while. You'd be amazed at all the people who have cooked dinner for our family since Matt passed away. I never knew we *knew* so many people! Some of the meals were okay but some of them . . . well, let's just say we'll all be thankful when Mom starts cooking again. Dad says she needs some rest after all that's happened. I hope the rest will make her feel better soon. I really miss my "before this happened" mom.

The good news is—tonight's meal will be yummy. Aunt Mandy makes awesome macaroni and cheese. Plus she'll bring my cousins Adam and Rebecca—they're Ben and Ricky's age—which will be fun for us kids. Maybe I should wipe off that Old Spice. Adam and Ben will definitely tease me because Ben knows the smell. Nah . . . I just feel like wearing it. It's kind of like keeping Matt with me.

Don't let my cousins open your pages. I will tuck you under my pillow.

Love ya,
Jessica

August 1
7:22 in the morning

Good morning D,

Just want to let you know how things turned out last night. The macaroni and cheese was delicious. Ben sniffed the Old Spice on me but he didn't tease me. It happened right when Aunt Mandy put a dish of steaming broccoli on the table.

Ben yelped, "What's that smell!?"

I calmly suggested, "It's the broccoli."

He giggled, "It's definitely not the broccoli—it's the spice!"

Aunt Mandy thought he was talking about a cooking spice, and she assured him she didn't use any spice in the dinner. I nervously used this "thumbs up" signal to Ben, which he knows means "I'll tell you later."

After dinner, I confessed the truth to him and Adam. Instead of making fun of me, they asked if they could wear some, too! Two minutes later Rebecca and Ricky bounced into the room and insisted we "share the spice!" Rebecca and Ricky didn't realize that deodorant is only supposed to go under the arms. They painted themselves with it! Luckily Aunt Mandy took the first whiff of us and hurried us into the shower before my mom could smell us. I doubt Mom would have smiled about it like Aunt Mandy did.

Aunt Mandy is a really great aunt.
That's all the news for now.

Love,
Jessie

August 2
6:45 at night

Dear Diary,

Today was one of those days when the youngest person in the Allman family discovered something very important. At lunchtime, Ricky stood up from his seat at the kitchen table and asked if it would be all right if he went out on the screen porch for a few minutes. Mom gets a little impatient with him when he doesn't sit still for meals but I think she understood the thoughtful expression on his face, and she gave him permission in a kitten quiet voice. He seemed to want his privacy so we tried to keep eating our peanut butter and jelly sandwiches as if he had never left the table. But we all secretly watched him looking up at the big oak trees in our yard, and we couldn't help but notice that he was talking to the trees in a voice even softer than a kitten's.

After a few minutes, he returned to the table and reported to us that he was just "asking G-d a few questions, just trying to find out if Matt was doing okay. Could G-d possibly give him back to us in a few days or . . . ."

I quickly interrupted Ricky because I thought he was about to make Mom cry. "Faye's coming tomorrow, Ricky. Let's talk about this with her."

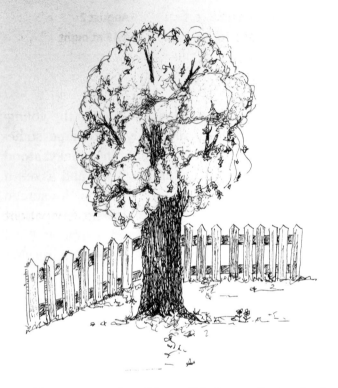

To my surprise, Mom didn't cry. Instead, she hugged Ricky and said, "Everyone in the family has lots of questions and sharing them is very important—even if we don't have the answers."

It made me feel good inside to see Mom giving Ricky a hug. I was also relieved to hear that it's good to share our questions. I have so many that pop in and out of my head all day. I hope Faye will have some answers tomorrow. I know Matt's not coming back but I wonder if she can tell us if he's okay.

We all seemed to feel a lot better after lunch, for some mysterious reason. Ben, Ricky and I were allowed to go under the sprinkler for two whole hours! It felt great!

Are you o.k.?

I'm ready for a good night's sleep. How about you?

Lots of love,
Jessica

August 3
7:36 at night

Dear Diary,

Faye came today a little bit before dinnertime. She wore this watch with rainbows on it that Ricky found fascinating. She was nice enough to let him wear it for most of our talk. She reminds me a little bit of my Grandma Ruth, has lots of love in her voice and some grey hair. Ricky blurted out his questions before she had even sat in her chair. "Can G-d give Matt back to our family in a few days? Is Matt doing okay? Can he see us from Heaven?"

Faye took a deep breath and sat motionless for what felt like hours. Then she slowly told Ricky that she understood how much he and all the family were missing Matt, but he could never be with us again in person, like really stand next to us or something, because his body doesn't work anymore.

"He can't breathe or eat or sleep or even feel hurt. But, Ricky, there's a *different* way he can be with you—and that's the 'inside of you way.'"

"The inside of me way?" Ricky asked, staring down at his belly.

"Well, yes, Ricky. Inside your thoughts. Like when you have a picture of him in your mind playing with you, or you can hear his laugh or even his voice when he was teasing you."

I looked over at Mom and Dad when she said this. Dad was staring at the floor and Mom suddenly looked at me, too. It's so hard to look at your mom when she's crying. I sat frozen as an icicle in my seat.

Luckily, Ben started making a big fuss before anyone could think for much longer. You see, his tooth went from being sort of loose to really loose and blood dripped down the finger he was jiggling the tooth with. Blood gives him the heebie-jeebies, and he's not shy about letting everyone know it. Next thing we knew, Faye offered to pull it out for him, and he was terrified but willing. He squeezed his eyes shut and opened his mouth wide as a cave. Diary, I never saw a grown-up yank a tooth out so calmly. She sure earned my respect!

Well Diary, I'm going to try hard to feel Matt inside of me. Right now I'm remembering his voice when he'd say "goodnight, Jessie." I can really, really remember that voice. I'm sure it's inside me forever. Maybe he'll be in my dreams tonight.

Love,
Jessie

August 4
7:49 at night

Dear Diary,

I wish I could personally thank the person who invented mail! Today I received another letter from Lindsay, and this time she included a picture she colored for me of the time we played weather station with her when she slept over during spring vacation. It's pretty difficult to invent a game that interests all the Allman kids *plus* a friend, but we did. In fact, Matt, being almost eleven years old, wasn't usually big on joining our games. On this sleepover, though, it was a stormy, blustery night, and we thought there might truly be a blackout or a flood. So we set up a weather station in my room with maps, a pretend t.v. camera, walkie talkies, and flashlights. We had a blast keeping track of the storm. One time the thunder was so explosive we all screamed and piled under my bed. Ricky claimed he smelled chocolate and next thing we knew Matt was passing around smooshed M&M's he'd been hiding in his pajama pocket. We have a strict "no food upstairs" policy in our house but it somehow felt okay to break the rules since it was Matt's idea.

Lindsay is a pretty good artist and she captured that sleepover memory amazingly well. Big deal if we all look a little more like Martians than people! She needs to improve the way she draws faces—but her M&M's are perfect! It was soooo thoughtful of her to make that for me.

I think I'll hang her drawing near my bed. On second thought, some people might get sad if they see it—like Mom or Dad. Maybe I'll keep it in my desk for now. It makes me a little sad, too. I miss Matt so much.

Goodnight, Diary.

Love,
Jessica

August 5
7:12 at night

Dear Diary,

I'm really excited to tell you about my day today. It was the first time in ages that each person in the Allman family, parents included, smiled. Quick smiles—yes; but they happened. Dad came home early from work. It was about 100 boiling degrees outside so Ben, Ricky and I were in bathing suits squirting each other with the garden hose in our backyard. Mom and Dad joined us in their bathing suits and offered to set up the sprinkler. We all took turns running through it and then we started playing this new game. Dad called out different groups to run through the water, like "girls!" (for me and Mom), "boys!" (for Dad, Ben and Ricky), "kids!," "parents!," and all sorts of fun combinations. There's something about running through a sprinkler that brings out the giggles and the sillies, and it felt so good to be that way with Mom and Dad. Sometimes in my mind I would say "Matt!" I tried to share the fun with him, too. It was a weird feeling to run with only two brothers instead of three when it was the "kids" turn. A lot of me felt happy because we were having so much fun. But part of me really missed Matt. I'm telling you this because I think it's important to let you know all my thoughts.

Well, I guess I wasn't the only one in the family missing Matt. At dinnertime Ricky asked if he could go to the screen porch for a few minutes. He started talking to the trees again, even waving his arms a little bit. When he returned to the kitchen table, he said, "I'm ready for dinner now. I just needed to ask G-d to tell Matt I pretended he was in my bathing suit pocket during our sprinkler game this afternoon."

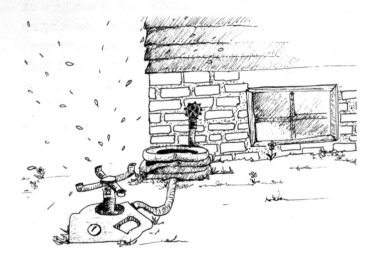

Leave it to Ricky to figure out a terrific way to keep Matt inside him! Faye would sure feel proud of him.

Sweet dreams,
Jessie

August 6
8:45 at night

Dear Diary,

This morning at breakfast Ben asked Mom if Dad would be home from work early enough to go with us under the sprinkler again. Mom said he'd be a little late tonight but maybe we could do it again another time. She suggested that Ben, Ricky and I pitch our camping tent in the backyard, and then we could bring games and snacks and books inside. We absolutely love setting up the tent and we hadn't done it yet this summer. Well, I'm sure you know why. But Mom's been acting a little more like Mom these past few days, which makes me feel so good inside. She used to be full of ideas for us when we ran out of things to do, but after Matt passed away, she needed a lot of rest and she stayed in bed more than a Mom usually would. So we kids really had to keep ourselves busy on our own. The tent idea was a great old-fashioned "Mom" idea. And luckily it was much cooler outside today than 100 boiling degrees.

Ben said something really smart to Mom at bedtime tonight. I'll tell you exactly how he said it because I can't say it any better. "Mom, it's lucky you had four children. It's very unlucky that one died but it's really lucky you still have three left."

It's strange how you can be very unlucky and lucky at the same time. I was supposed to be reading in my bed when they were saying goodnight, but I overheard Ben and I got Ricky out of bed and ran into Ben's room to give everybody a big hug. Diary, I'm a little lucky, too, because I have great brothers. Matt is inside of me and Ben and Ricky are by my side.

Well, it's super late because we were in the tent until dark with flashlights, so I'm signing off for now. I'm lucky to have you, too!

Love,
Jessica

August 7

7:17 at night

Dear D,

It's amazing how one day can feel so different from the day that came before it. We kept the tent up today but Ben didn't want to play in it for too long. He was in a blah mood because his favorite baseball tee-shirt that used to be Matt's, got a really big hole in it. He felt sad that something special to Matt got ruined. I don't blame him. I wish I could've fixed it for him but it was more of a huge rip than a fixable hole.

When it was time for showers tonight, Ben just started crying and crying. Luckily, Dad had come home early from work so after Ben put on his pajamas, Dad sat down with him and helped him write a list of ways to make himself feel better during really sad moods like today's. I was kind of amazed, Diary, because Dad actually sat at Matt's desk to make the list! Not only did he sit in Matt's chair, but he opened some drawers to find paper and a pencil! His heart didn't freeze or anything, but I did notice that he kept the drawer open a little longer than usual, and he shielded his eyes with his hand, as if it were too sunny in the room. Once he had the supplies, though, he took his hand away from his eyes and got right down to business. I wonder what else was in those drawers, Diary. If only I could be like my dad, and just convince myself I'm looking for something, for paper and a pencil, let's say. This way I can have a look, but not a terribly long look, and then maybe I'll feel better, and I'll have a few more of Matt's things to remember him by. I think I could handle it, but only if it were a quick look, Diary.

Well, let me tell you about the list Ben and Dad put together. Ben was nice enough to call a kids' meeting so he could share some ideas with Ricky and me. I was really glad he did because I'm sure these will help me sometimes. I'll share the list with you, too. They came up with some really helpful thoughts.

Believe it or not "Cry" was the number one suggestion! I think crying feels awful while you're doing it, but afterwards you usually do feel more okay about things. Weird, huh? Here's the rest of the list:

2. Write in my diary.
3. Give someone a hug.
4. Talk to someone close to me and tell them how I feel.
5. Talk about things that make me happy.
6. Read books.
7. Draw a picture of a "Matt" memory.
8. Look at a photograph of Matt, especially Matt's smile.
9. Think about Mom and Dad and that Mom and Dad love me very much.

10. Think about the whole family. I decided to add this: Especially Ricky when he wakes up in the morning and has pointy hair.
11. At night, imagine something happy and then try to dream about it.

I know the one about Ricky works, and the one about you works, too. You're the best diary ever!

Love,
Jessie

August 8
5:27 before dinner

Dear Diary,

School will be starting in a few weeks, which gives me a creepy crawly spider feeling in my stomach. I'm just not ready to be a fourth grader without my big brother. I wish time could move backwards; I wish there could be a rewind button or a backspace button or some powerful button to get my whole family back to June. Okay Jessie, think happier thoughts. Remember how much Matt loved school. He was practically a nerd!

Well, at least there will be one sort of good part about starting school, and that's because of this cool family project invented by my mom that we worked on in the backyard today. It has something to do with school, something to do with having many empty baskets sitting on shelves in our basement, and a lot to do with remembering Matt. We have heaps of empty baskets around the house because our family received many generous deliveries of food from neighbors after Matt passed away. The baskets definitely cheered us up, and made sure we remembered to eat.

Mom decided that we should preserve one basket made of plain straw as a way to remember how nice people have been to us during our sad time. And since Matt really loved school and—don't ask me why or how—enjoyed doing his homework, we could create a homework basket filled with all the supplies we would need for assignments, like crayons, glue, pencils, rulers—that kind of stuff. The really great part was that every person in the family could help paint the basket with words or pictures that had something to do with Matt; the basket would be a "Matt Homework Basket."

Our backyard became a family art studio! Mom covered our picnic table with newspaper and filled two art palettes with every color of paint imaginable. She laid out lots of paint brushes, thick and thin, and we the Allman family became the Artistic family. The best part was we didn't need smocks. It was 95 semi-boiling degrees today so all five of us worked in bathing suits and we sprayed ourselves clean with the hose when we were completely finished. Ricky looked like a painting himself by the time he was done. He's not the neatest artist you'll ever meet.

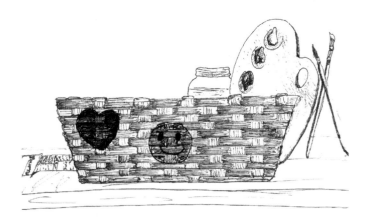

Anyhow, here are some of the designs we thought of for the basket: Ricky painted a smiley face and a red heart. Ben painted a basketball and a computer. I painted a baseball and another red heart. Mom painted a pad and a pen. Dad painted a cup of lemonade and a chocolate chip cookie. Mom and Dad were in charge of painting any words we wanted to include to describe Matt. It was really hard to paint neat letters onto a bumpy basket, but they did a fine job. Here are some of the words we included: good sport, good friend, poet, sensitive, funny, creative, brave and loving.

Some of us Allmans are less artistic than others. Dad's chocolate chip cookie looks more like a meatloaf. But I think the basket came out terrific. Maybe it will help me to do a better job on my homework. Maybe it will help me face going back to school. I think Matt would be proud of his family.

Tomorrow when the paint is dry, I'll keep you inside the basket for a little while so you can check it out!

Friends always,
Jessica

August 9
7:39 at night

Dear Diary,

I think making the "Matt Homework Basket" yesterday gave me the jitters about school. I do have a few weeks left so I guess I'll try not to think about it too much. I keep imagining tons of kids staring at me in the cafeteria and whispering to each other. Worse yet, I hope nobody will *dare* to ask me about it. I can talk with Lindsay about Matt because I can talk about anything with Lindsay; in fact I feel better when I talk about things with Lindsay. But kids I don't know very well? No way! Oh Diary, going back to school is going to be very difficult.

You wouldn't believe what Ben blabbered today. We were playing at our neighbor's, the Gilmans, who have four children. But today there were six Gilman children because two cousins were visiting. All of a sudden I hear Ben telling Joey, one of the cousins, that his brother died, and he told him exactly how it happened. Joey looked like he'd just seen a ghost fly across the backyard.

When we were walking home, I gave Ben a piece of my mind. "I would never tell people what happened to Matt. It's really private and it's nobody else's business. Joey Gilman! What does Joey Gilman need to know for?"

His answer? "Jessica, I don't think it has to be a secret. Why should it be a secret? He was our brother!"

What do you think, Diary? Don't you think what happened to Matt should be kept—maybe not secret—but private? I sure wish you could write me back sometimes. This is *really* bothering me. I think I will ask Faye her opinion about this when we see her again. She's coming to visit us tomorrow night. I can understand talking about Matt with people I'm close to. But why would I tell the Gilman's cousin about it? Ben is crazy!

Hopefully, I'll have more information for you tomorrow.

Joey Gilman sticks out his tongue and screams bad words when he loses a game! I would never tell him anything about my family!

It's been a long day.

Love,
Jessica

August 10
7:41 at night

Dear Diary,

Did you know that if someone dies in your family, there's no need to keep it a secret because it's not something to be ashamed of? At least according to Faye it's not. I guess Ben and me were both sort of right on this one because as Faye said tonight, "It's perfectly o.k. to talk about Matt's death to others *if* you feel like you want to. There's no right or wrong decision, it just depends on what *feels* right to *you*."

I'll tell you one thing. It feels mad hard for *me* to talk about it.

But she kind of helped me understand why. I guess I wanted to keep Matt's death a secret from people because I almost feel like an oddball or sort of ashamed. No other kids I know had such a bad thing happen to their family. I'm not like regular kids, anymore, Diary. But Faye made a very good point. "People should only feel shame if they do something wrong like lie or cheat or steal. But experiencing a death in the family is a very sad event that has *absolutely nothing* to do with *doing* something wrong, and that's why you shouldn't feel like it needs to be a secret."

In my mind her point makes sense, but I can't exactly make my feelings magically disappear. I think those feelings may have shrunk—but they haven't completely disappeared yet. That seems impossible.

Speaking of magic, you'll never guess who's in my doorway right now wearing a magician's hat, pajamas that actually have a bunny tail on the tushy, ready with wand and handkerchief to do a bedtime trick for me. You guessed it—tricky Ricky. Just in time, really! The only problem is I'll never get to bed. When Ricky does magic he insists on repeating the same trick again and again. Diary, he's not a very talented magician. Cute, but definitely not talented.

Wish me luck,
Jessica

August 11
7:19 at night

Dear Diary,

Today I was cleaning up my room trying to get things organized for when I go back to school. Especially my desk—what a mess! I found these red heart sticker earrings at the bottom of my desk drawer, the kind that look just like pierced earrings except you don't need pierced ears to wear them because they stick like glue to your ears. Aunt Mandy gave them to me for my fourth birthday and they reminded me of a really funny Matt story, which I think I should tell you so we can both always remember it.

One day Mom had to go out for a zillion errands, so she asked our babysitter Annie to come for a little while. I decided to dress-up for Annie in my favorite red sparkle dress from my princess Halloween costume, gold party shoes and of course my new cool earrings from Aunt Mandy. I was dancing around the house showing off my outfit to everyone when Matt bumped into me and an earring slipped into my ear. He saw it slip in and vanish, and called Annie to see if she could fish it out. She could see it inside my ear but it was too deep for her to remove it.

When Mom came home she called our pediatrician and he informed her that we had to go to an ear specialist. Apparently, a heart-shaped sticker earring embedded in the ear can hurt your hearing. Matt begged to come along because he felt like the whole thing was his fault, which it sort of was because he did bump into me and my earring. The doctor wanted to poke around in my ear with this nasty looking instrument and I plain refused to let him touch me. I figured I could still hear (not as well as usual but well enough), earring or no earring, so why not just leave it in there for decoration! Matt tried to show me that the doctor wouldn't hurt me. He acted really brave and said "Doctor, look in my ear with that instrument so Jessie can see that it doesn't hurt me and it won't hurt her." The doctor went along with his idea except the doctor discovered gobs and gobs of earwax in Matt's ear that he thought should be removed. Matt looked a little nervous but he said it would be okay to take it out. Next thing I knew Matt was squirming in pain but still trying to be brave in front of me. Then I started to feel guilty that I got him into *his* mess so I let the doctor pluck out the earring.

We used to laugh a lot about that story together. I think I'll stick the earrings I found today on this page as a special decoration. Hope you like it!

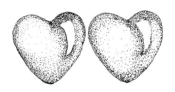

You know, Diary, it's amazing that one little thing found by accident in *my* desk drawer cooked up a gigantic, wacky, very special memory. There must be a treasure box of stuff like that inside Matt's desk. When I feel like *my* heart's a little stronger I'm going to see for myself!

Love,
Jessica

August 13
7:45 at night

Dear Diary,

I forgot to tell you that my brothers and I were having a sleepover at my Grandparents' house last night. I completely forgot to pack you in my overnight bag, so that's why I didn't write yesterday. We had a pretty fun time. Grandma Ruth and Grandpa Meyer always let us stay up extra late and eat big ice cream sundaes before bed (at home we're only allowed to have a slice of apple before bed. . . which my mom says is better for our teeth and sweeter for our dreams). They took us to their town beach for the day, but they were really strict about our swimming. We weren't allowed to swim waist deep in the waves like we would have if my parents had been with us (although my parents won't take us anywhere near the water these days). We could only be in the water ankle deep! Grandpa had a really serious look on his face when he told us the swimming rules, and we didn't dare try to negotiate with him like we would for later bed times or an extra scoop of ice cream.

I know he was remembering Matt. I sure was. The last time we had been to the beach was with Matt. I remember how Ben, Ricky and I had covered Matt with sand from his toes to his belly (he was lounging in the sand giggling because Ricky kept tickling him but he still didn't budge from his sand trap). Finally, he was so tickle-tortured he broke free and started chasing Ricky in the sand. Then a seagull pooped on Ricky and everybody laughed (except Ricky who started to cry because everyone was laughing at him). Yesterday, I was trying to figure out which spot on the beach was the one where we had played together. I actually think I found it, and I made a heart out of shells in the sand where I thought it was.

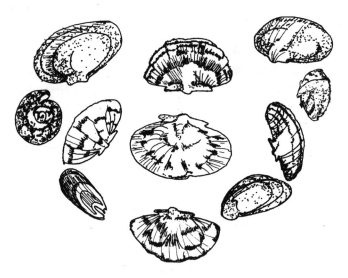

I wish Matt could know I'm thinking of him. Well, you know I'm thinking of him, Diary, and I guess that's a start. Thanks for listening.

Love,
Jessie

August 14
7:49 at night

Dear Diary,

Today was a "Good Things Happened in the Allman Family" day! Hooray for August 14th! Well, it was a pretty simple summer day—no major occasion or anything—but let me tell you why it was so special. It started with Mom making us yummy waffles for breakfast. Then Aunt Mandy drove me, Ben and Ricky to her town pool for the day. We played Marco Polo with Adam and Rebecca in this giant pool that's especially fun because it has no deep end so all of us could stand anywhere in the pool. (Do you know how to play Marco Polo? It's sort of like a pool game version of hide and seek except you use your ears to figure out where someone's hiding instead of your eyes.)

At the end of the day, Mom and Dad met us at Aunt Mandy's for a barbecue and it felt very special to have our family and Aunt Mandy's family together, especially because it was the first time our whole family had been out together since Matt passed away. Mom and Dad haven't wanted to go out much since Matt passed away but they seemed okay tonight about going to Aunt Mandy's.

Guess what Ricky announced at Aunt Mandy's dinner table? First, you need to know that his fifth birthday is tomorrow. Well, after three bites of hot dog, he stood up on his chair and said, "Mom and

Dad . . . I want swimming lessons for my birthday present." I thought Mom and Dad might freak out about Ricky's wanting to spend more time in the water because of what happened to Matt. But they said they thought it was a great idea and Mom said she'd call the Town Recreation Center tomorrow to inquire.

I'm really proud of Ricky because he's very brave. I already know how to swim but I'm not sure how I'd feel about it if I *didn't* know how. When your big brother loses his life in the water, that's a gigantic scary thing. I guess it's really important for Ricky to learn to swim but I think he's a brave and smart guy to suggest it himself—and as a birthday present! Gosh, I would be hoping for electric trains or something!

I'm sleepy. . .

Love,
Jessica

August 15
8:11 at night

Dear Diary,

I'm stuffed! We had a huge spaghetti and ice cream cake dinner for Ricky's birthday and I think I should have skipped those last few spoonfuls. I have to say it didn't feel as happy as the usual Allman birthday celebration but we had a little fun.

Ben and I made a beautiful butterfly habitat in a big clear plastic container filled with grass and flowers for Ricky's present. We were able to include three gorgeous butterflies we caught for him. We usually have no luck catching butterflies but today—it was amazing—we caught three really colorful ones. I imagined in my mind that somehow Matt sent those butterflies for Ricky's birthday. Crazy, huh? That's a secret thought between you and me, okay?

At cake time Ricky blew out his candles and wished his wish (out loud, of course; Ricky has been making out loud wishes since he learned the English language. He's not the most private kid you'll ever meet). I'm sure you can guess what his wish was: "I wish I could ride my birthday balloons to the sky and see my big brother Mattie!" The kitchen sure became quiet after that wish. I couldn't even look Mom and Dad's way.

Quiet never lasts for long in our house, though. About two seconds later Ricky proceeded to spill his milk on Ben. Ben hates to be the victim of a spill, particularly a milk spill, and he lets you know loud and clear how he feels about it. Although I must say, I think he took it a little better than usual, maybe because he didn't want to spoil Ricky's wish.

I wonder if we'll find any butterflies tomorrow.

Sweet dreams,
Jessica

August 16
5:30 before dinner

Dear Diary,

Sometimes it feels like everywhere I go, I bump into a reminder of Matt. I kind of want to think about him but it also gives me a bad feeling because I miss him so, so much. In the afternoon Mom took us to our favorite store, Big Top. Big Top has every toy, candy and school supply imaginable. It's usually really fun to go there because no matter what important thing we need, like notebooks or glue or poster board, we're usually allowed to pick a treat like gum or a lollipop or candy bar. I spend a good part of my allowance at Big Top!

Today was the first time in my life that I couldn't wait to escape from there. We were choosing lunch boxes for school and none of them looked as exciting as they did in past years. I was just about to announce that I wouldn't need one this year, that home schooling would be a far better choice for me, when all of a sudden we saw Andy Alper, Marc Clare and Steve Buck, three of Matt's friends buying candy. They were extremely nice to us and even bought bubblegum for me, Ben and Ricky. But I just kept staring at them and picturing Matt with them eating sour suckers (his favorite candy in the world, which I think is awful because it's so sour you feel like your mouth will burst). Mom hardly spoke to us when we drove home. She wasn't mad

or anything but she must've been silently picturing Matt eating sour suckers with his friends, too.

I didn't know what to say to her but when we
got out of the car I ran over to her and gave her
a record-setting heartbeat to heartbeat hug. Faye
was sure right about hugs! They're better than any
medicine.

Love ya,
Jessica

P.S. We didn't see any pretty butterflies today.

August 17
7:53 at night

Dear Diary,

It must be "See Matt's Friends Week" or something. I told you about the Big Top episode yesterday. Well, today Scott Anderson, Mattie's best friend, rang our doorbell. (Remember I told you about the picture of Matt and Scott that Ben taped next to his pillow? He's the Scott I'm writing about.) He just returned home from a baseball overnight camp and he stopped by to give us brownies his mom had baked and to see how our family was doing. To tell you the truth, he didn't look like he was doing so well when he walked into our house. He's usually really bouncy—or at least he's bouncing some kind of ball which makes him *seem* bouncy— but today he was spider quiet and he didn't stay for too long, probably because he felt so weird being in our house without Matt. Ricky and Ben usually tackle him and perform their day's quota of wrestling when he's over. But today . . . no way! We all stood around like trees.

Finally Mom insisted he come to the kitchen and have some brownies and lemonade with us, which he did. And Ricky, as usual, got all of us to crack a smile when he sneezed a monstrous sneeze in the middle of chewing his brownie. You can imagine how quickly we slid our seats away from him at that moment!

It feels sort of good to see Matt's friends because I almost feel like Matt's in the next room or something. Maybe it's another way of keeping Matt inside of us. I think Faye would agree, don't you?

She's coming tomorrow. I bet we'll have a lot to talk about.

Love ya,
Jessie

August 18
5:24 before dinner

Dear Diary,

I think it's about time to start an official count-down toward the day Lindsay comes home from her Grandma's country house. (I've decided to forget that school starts soon after that. So, Diary, please, don't remind me.) One more week until I can see my bff. I can barely wait! You're a great friend, Diary, but I sure will be happy to be with Lindsay Beth Silber once again.

Faye came to our house today and we talked for awhile about what it feels like to see Matt's friends. I explained that when we saw Andy, Marc and Steve in Big Top, and then Scott Anderson yesterday, I felt bombarded by a trillion feelings, and I needed to make a quick exit. I've always liked Matt's friends so the old me was glad to see them and happy about the treats they gave my brothers and me. But the new me (the one whose brother passed away) felt dark and empty inside because Matt was missing from their group. I couldn't even tell Faye and the family a very private secret that I'll tell you, Diary. The new me felt really worried about my Mom's feelings when *she* looked at Matt's friends. If it was tough for me, it must've been triple awful for her. Anyhow, Faye explained that it's okay to feel partly good about an event and partly bad about an event because it's just a natural reaction to the way things are for our family. Feelings are not right or wrong but they can be jumbled up when we've lost someone we love very much. She understood why I felt like running out of Big Top. It just doesn't feel very comfortable when so many feelings happen at once so I needed to escape from that uncomfortable feeling.

After Faye explained all that, Mom shared something that made me smile. She said that my "after Big Top hug" brightened her afternoon a whole lot. Maybe I have a little bit of Ricky's "make people smile" talent.

Mom is calling us downstairs for dinner now.

Your friend,
Jessica

August 19
7:46 at night

Dear Diary,

Six more days until L.B.S. comes home. I'm really excited about that but I'm really nervous that school is getting closer. It's hard to imagine standing at our bus stop with just three Allman kids. Maybe Mom will start driving us to school instead. Maybe I should find out more about being homeschooled. I doubt Mom would let me do that. Besides, I guess I would miss Lindsay.

Today it rained so Ben, Ricky and I held a kid's meeting to figure out good games to play. Ben invented a new game that was pretty cool called "The Helping Office." We set up a desk in the family room with paper, pencils, our sticker collection and other office supplies, and we took turns being the helpers and being the customer with a problem.

When it was Ben's turn, he said he was afraid he'd sleep late on the first day of school because Matt wouldn't be there to wake him up like he used to do. He was pretty panicked that he'd miss the bus. Ricky and I wrote out a promise to wake him up extra early so he'd have plenty of time to get ready. (Actually, I wrote the words and Ricky illustrated with pictures and stickers.) Ricky loves to play the helper. You can tell he takes it very seriously because when it's his turn he puts on his doctor's costume complete with stethoscope and first aid kit, even though our office was more for worries in your mind, not for sore throats or ear infections or anything.

Diary, I also admitted to Ben that I had been wondering whether I could step onto the bus without Matt. For a second we were both laughing about Matt's bodyguard skills—he protected us like no other—but then we both became mouse quiet and thoughtful. Ben and I made a pact to sit together on the first day and walk as far as we could together to our classroom. He's a good guy that Ben. Maybe if we stick together we'll be okay.

I almost forgot to tell you! Mom even played with us for a little while! We helped her figure out a list of our favorite lunchbox menus for school. We can be pretty picky people when it comes to school lunch but with the menus we made I think we'll avoid starvation. Peanut butter and marshmallow fluff sandwiches are my absolute favorite, but Mom only allows us to have fluff for lunch on our birthday.

It's kind of fun to work with partners and do problem-solving. Maybe going back to school will be o.k. after all. I hope kids will still want to be my partner. Who knows what they'll think about a girl whose brother passed away. Lindsay would be my partner no matter what, but I doubt we'll be in the same class. I'm ready to snooze, Diary.

Love ya,
Dr. Jessica

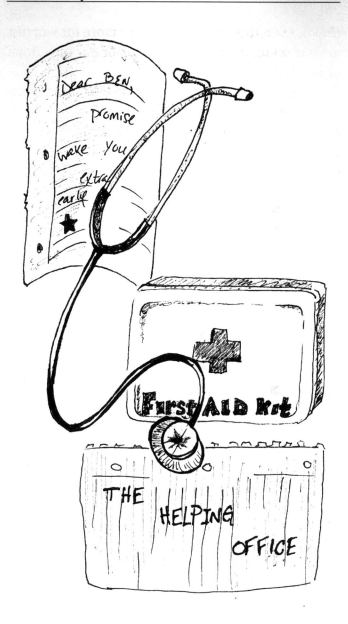

August 20
7: 49 at night

Dear D,

Yesterday's problems were so much simpler to solve than today's problems. The day started out really great because Mom decided we could picnic in the backyard for breakfast. It was a deliciously warm summer morning when you could go outside right after a shower and let your hair dry in the sun. Ricky and I helped Mom set up our special picnic blanket spread with two trays of breakfast food and extra orange juice so we wouldn't have to keep running inside for refills.

Ben didn't feel like helping with setup, so he sat and watched us with a gloomy look on his face. During the picnic he wasn't eating much but when he rejected a jelly doughnut (Ben usually eats three at a time), Mom asked him what was wrong.

At first he said, "Nothing, nothing, nothing!" Then a few minutes later he said, "Well, actually, something *is* wrong, but I don't want to tell anybody." Then a few minutes later, he blurted out, "Just tell me the truth about one thing: if something really bad happened to someone in your family, does that mean something really bad will happen to you?" Of course he didn't mention Matt's name but we all got the point. He didn't have to explain any further to me because that question had also been on my mind, but I was afraid to ask anybody for an answer. Even you, Diary! SORRY!

Mom moved closer to Ben and she put her arm around him. She sat very still for awhile and then she answered him in a very soft voice. She explained that what happened to Matt was really, really rare and really, really unusual. Most kids do all the regular kid stuff like school and summer camp, biking, playing, swimming. Nothing really bad happens to them. In fact, they have lots of fun. Then they grow up to be Moms and Dads, even Grandmas and Grandpas. She tried to reassure him that he'd be a Grandpa someday and do all the fun, growing up stuff in between. (Grandpa Ben, can you imagine that? How about Grandpa Ricky? Ricky will still be spilling milk in his old age, I'm sure of it!) He seemed to feel a little better once he'd shared that big worry. Actually, I felt better, too! I should've at least written to you about it, Diary. Today was perfect proof that it's not good to keep big worries inside. Worries are not meant to be lonely, I guess; they need to be shared.

The official countdown continues . . . five more days until Lindsay comes home. Wow!

Love ya,
The future Grandma Jessie

August 21
7:52 at night

Dear Diary,

Today I felt a little bit like Ricky because I found myself . . . not talking to the trees, but close! After lunch Ben and Ricky were busy watching a TV show that I don't like so I decided to go out in the backyard with a blanket and a book and just relax. I parked myself beneath the big oak trees that Ricky likes to talk to, and I lay under them watching green leaves sway and admiring the beautiful lace roof they formed over my head.

When I see beautiful things in nature I feel like G-d is close by. At that moment under the trees I looked hard up at the sky, I'm not sure why. Maybe I was hoping to see G-d's face or Matt's smile in a cloud. Nothing appeared, of course. I simply felt very peaceful under that tree. And I guess I can believe that this was because Matt and G-d *were* somehow close by. They were in my heart at least, right Diary?

With love,
Jessica

August 22
8:07 at night

Dear Diary,

Today Grandma Ruth and Grandpa Meyer came over to visit. They took me, Ben and Ricky to buy our back-to-school sneakers. I really didn't want to buy new shoes this year but I didn't have the heart to disappoint Grandma and Grandpa so I chose the same sneakers as last year. It was very sad finishing so quickly in the shoe store. When Matt was alive, he would try on nearly every shoe before he would make a decision. He would drive all of us crazy because he could never choose something until at least pair number ten. Today we just picked our sneakers without any fuss and before we knew it, we were deciding where to go for lunch. I never thought it would feel terrible when an Allman kids' shopping trip went smoothly. But, Diary, it felt terrible.

Maybe I should become a fussy sneaker shopper just to put a little bit of Matt back into the event. I think that's an excellent idea! Next time I will try on at least ten pairs of sneakers before even considering the pair I really want! I wish I had thought of this earlier.

Three more days until Lindsay comes home (I forgot to record the countdown in yesterday's journal entry). That's a good bedtime thought!

Love,
Jessie

August 23
8:30 at night

Dear Diary,

Fifteen years ago today my parents got married. So you know what that makes today? Their wedding anniversary. The day almost passed without any of us kids even knowing it was their anniversary until Aunt Mandy appeared at our front door at 6:30 p.m. to inform all of us (including my parents!) that she'd be babysitting for us so my parents could go on a date on their special day.

The weird thing was . . . my parents *didn't* want to go out but we kids *wanted* them to go. Usually (usually means before Matt passed away) we'd have protested that it wasn't fair to leave us home but this time we practically locked them out of the house. We desperately wanted to see our mom and dad smile and have fun together, and it didn't seem very nice of them to refuse Aunt Mandy's offer. After all, she had gone to the trouble of finding a sitter for Adam and Rebecca so she could take care of us. Finally, they agreed to go for a quick dinner but they must be the only parents on this earth who look depressed, even annoyed, when a surprise babysitter shows up so they can go out together. Oh well. I guess it's hard to do fun things when you're sad. Maybe once they arrived at the restaurant, they started to enjoy themselves a little.

I felt Matt inside of me a lot tonight because I did some of the stuff he usually did when a baby-sitter came, like tuck in Ben and calm Ricky down when he couldn't fall asleep because he missed Mom and Dad. Matt used to tell Ricky the sooner he fell asleep, the sooner he'd see Mom and Dad because morning would come and then they'd be back home.

Aunt Mandy said I was a great helper. I wish I could thank Matt for helping me be a great helper. Well,

Matt . . . wherever you are . . . thanks big brother!

L.B.S. comes home in two more days. Awesome!

With love,
Jessica

August 24
8:42 at night

Dear D,

If I sound more cheerful than yesterday, there's a very good reason why. When a person's best friend comes home a day early after being away all summer, that person is likely to feel monkey happy. And that person is me!

Lindsay surprised us today after lunch and stayed until way after dinner. Actually, you sort of met her, Diary, because I let her read some of your pages. She thought you were terrific! In fact, she's going to start a diary, too.

Even Ben and Ricky were happy to see her. When she arrived, we were actually in the middle of making her a huge "Welcome Home Lindsay" sign decorated with chocolate kisses. I have to admit that I used to get annoyed sometimes when Ben and Ricky would butt in on my playtime with Lindsay, but today I felt glad to share her with them (for part of the time, anyway!). I guess we all missed Matt being around and we needed to stick together.

The sort of best part of our visit was when all four of us had a giant pillow fight. I laughed so hard I almost peed in my pants (oops!). We were pillow fighting in Ben and Matt's room when I knew I couldn't hold it in any more. Lucky for me the bathroom is right across the hall from their bedroom. It was a close call but I made a mad dash and made it just in time. When the pillow fight was over we each claimed a pillow and relaxed for a couple of minutes on the carpet. I found myself staring at the ceiling and feeling suddenly guilty about having so much fun in Matt's room without Matt. Judging by how quiet all four of us suddenly became, I'll bet I wasn't the only one feeling like a creep.

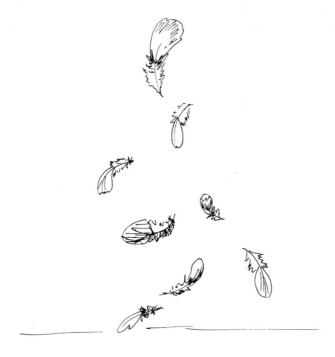

I think I need Faye's advice on this. It's crazy but having fun is not as fun as it used to be. Faye visits tomorrow so I'll try to explain this to her.

Friends always,
Jessie

August 25
8:03 at night

Dear Diary,

I think Faye's visit today was very successful.
It started out with a very nice treat: she baked our
family a delicious zucchini bread with vegetables
she grew in her garden. At first Ben and Ricky were
holding their noses when she offered them a slice
because they think vegetables and anything made
with vegetables are pewy. I elbowed them to remind
them of polite manners and they politely agreed to
have a taste, and they actually liked it because it
was actually major yummy.

After that snack, Faye asked us how things were
going and I answered they were going okay, so long
as things weren't too fun because it felt sort of bad
to have any fun. Faye looked really worried when I
said that. Come to think of it . . . Mom and Dad did,
too. There was total silence for a long minute and
then Faye asked if anything special had happened
to make me feel that way, so I told her all about
the pillow fight last night and how sad I felt after-
ward. She told me my feeling was a really important
one to share because it would be easier to handle
if I understood why the feeling was happening. And
here's why, Diary: because why should I have fun
if Matt can't have fun? That's how my heart feels. I
guess that's how Mom and Dad's heart felt on their
anniversary, too. Faye's view is that Matt wouldn't

want me or anyone in the family to stop living because of his passing. She reminded us that living means experiencing good times, too.

According to Faye, and I strongly agree with her, if we're going to keep Matt inside of us, then the real Matt was about good times; he wasn't about sadness and sitting around. We want to carry the real, life-loving Matt with us each day. Diary, my mind knows Faye is right but I guess it's hard to convince my *heart* that it's okay to have fun. It's worth trying, though. And it's good to know I'm not a completely crazy nine-year- old girl who thinks it's sad to have fun.

Well, I will be sure to have a fun day tomorrow.

Happy Dreams,
Jessica

August 26
7:00 at night

Dear Diary,

I guess we can't always plan fun days. As much as I wanted today to be a fun day, I found it nearly impossible to have fun on the day before a new school year begins, especially a school year that will happen without my oldest brother. From the minute the mail came early in the morning, and Mom opened the letters about our teacher and room assignments, I had bats flying in my stomach nonstop. I wish school years could just start in the middle so we wouldn't have to experience all the nervousness of opening day. Maybe I shouldn't be nervous because probably nobody will talk to me anyway because they won't know what to say to a girl whose brother passed away over the summer. At least I know Lindsay will talk to me, and the really great news is . . . Lindsay and I have the same teacher for the first time ever! So if kids look at me funny, at least I can count on Lindsay for support.

The other major good part of this whole situation is I have Mrs. Lindner for my teacher this year and she's one of the nicest teachers in the school. At least that was Matt's opinion. He never had her but some of his friends did and he spent all of fourth grade wishing he could switch teachers. I wish I could tell him that an Allman kid finally got Mrs. Lindner for a teacher. Ben was assigned to Mr.

Douglas who's an awesome second grade teacher. He does really fun projects and has really fun parties, and . . . the word is he never yells. Ben's really happy that he's in his class . . . but he's still worried about sleeping late and missing the bus. (If you're wondering why I'm writing to you so early in the evening it's because we have to go to bed extra early tonight so we won't have any trouble getting ready for school in the morning.)

I think Ricky is the guy who's most prepared for school even though he doesn't start kindergarten for another twelve months. He packed a backpack with markers, paper, snacks and toys and he left it by the front door so he'd be ready for our first day of school. I hope he doesn't have a fit when he finds out that he doesn't come into our classrooms with us. How embarrassing would that be!

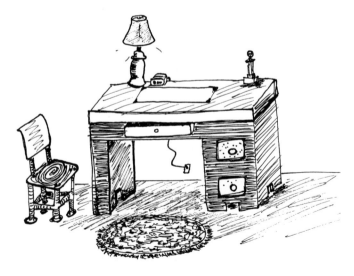

Diary, I'm going to tell you something that nobody else knows. When I was getting my backpack ready, I really wanted to tuck something of Matt's inside of it. Nothing big, just a pen or ruler or something. I actually sat at his desk for a couple of minutes when Ben was in the shower and tried to convince my hands to open a drawer. I was really close to opening it, Diary, but I lost my chance because when Ben finished his shower he wasn't too happy to find me snooping around his room. Oh well. Maybe I can try again another time. I'm getting braver about it, Diary. And it would be really nice to have something of Matt's with me everyday.

Truthfully, I'm not the least bit sleepy but I think I'll sign off for now and read for a little while. I'm sure I'll have lots to write to you about after tomorrow. Wish me luck!

Your fourth grade friend,
Jessie

August 27

7:12 at night

Dear Diary,

Well, I made it through the first day of school, and gosh do I feel relieved! The bats have flown out of my stomach, thank goodness, because they were driving me crazy. Mrs. Lindner is even nicer than Matt said she was. She gave each of us a "welcome pencil set" with our names painted on the pencil case, and she brought in special homemade M&M cookies for our first class snack of the year. She let us choose our own seats for the first few days of class until she gets to know us better and decides where our permanent seat should be. That was an especially fabulous situation for me because I was able to sit next to Lindsay Beth Silber. Actually, Diary, the kids were really nice to me today and only one boy, William Kingsley, stared at me as if I had purple eyes and orange hair. (I ignored him.) Andrew and Jeff (remember those nursery school "Dads" I told you about?) came up to me during lunchtime and said they were sorry about Matt, which really shocked me. It's not like they went on and on about it for too long, but they said just enough to make me feel okay being around kids again.

I had a surprise lunch today! It's a wonder anybody wanted to sit next to me after they discovered what was in my lunchbox! Mom must've been having the first day of school jitters, too, because instead of sticking the foil package from the refrigerator that contained my peanut butter and banana sandwich into my lunchbox, she grabbed the foil package that contained a piece of uncooked salmon and put that in my lunchbox. It was a bit hard to keep this mishap a secret because, ugh . . . what a smell! I ended up buying cafeteria pizza for lunch but I have to pay back the cashier tomorrow. So much for all the time Ben, Ricky and I spent creating lunch menus for Mom during our "Helping Office" game.

Diary, Mom was mouse quiet today and her eyes had that watery look. I know she must've been sad sending only two of us back to school. It's good Ricky doesn't go to kindergarten until next year. He's very good company for her. Today he presented Mom with a frog he caught in the backyard. Ben and I weren't home yet, but I'm guessing Mom wasn't mouse quiet at that moment.

I'm feeling pretty sleepy, Diary. I'll be back tomorrow night with more scoop.

Love ya lots,
Jessica

August 28
7:28 at night

Dear Diary,

School was going pretty well today, until about an hour after lunch when I felt like I needed a genie to help me disappear for a little while. You know how at the beginning of the school year teachers have you do these "getting to know you" types of activities? Well, Mrs. Lindner has a tradition of making "All About Me" posters with her students, which for most kids would be really fun because you get to use all the class art supplies when they're brand new, like markers and sparkle glue and glitter and sequins. You make a big poster that celebrates who you are and you include your hobbies, your favorite color, your favorite food, a person you admire, and. . .here's the hard part . . . information about your family, like how many brothers and sisters you have. I took a big gulp when I saw the part about family but I decided I would definitely include Matt on my poster because he would always be my brother, even if he weren't here anymore.

Everything would've been just fine if this know-it-all girl in my class, Olivia Michaels, didn't look over my shoulder at my work and try to correct my information. "Jessica, you don't have three brothers anymore." Can you *believe* she said that? I must've turned Martian green because Mrs. Lindner came right over and pointed out some areas on Olivia's poster that still needed work, and she took me into the hallway to get a drink of water. She actually hugged me and apologized for Olivia's hurtful comment, and tried to explain that Olivia didn't mean to hurt my feelings. I wondered to myself what the heck Olivia meant to do if not to hurt my feelings but I didn't say much back to Mrs. Lindner because my eyes were burning and I also felt like Ricky's frog was caught in my throat, blocking up my voice.

Well, that was enough of fourth grade for me today. I wasn't about to go back to my desk with a crybaby look on my face. I asked Mrs. Lindner if I could go to the nurse for a little while and I was kind of surprised that she let me go. Actually, she escorted me there and had a few whispers with the nurse before she went back to class. The nurse didn't even ask me what was wrong but she offered me a cherry ice pop, which I decided to accept and by the time I finished that, it was time to go home.

I guess I'm lucky that Olivia waited to be a mean blabbermouth until the end of the day. But what will I do tomorrow? How can I bear to walk back into Mrs. Lindner's room? I definitely should've asked to be homeschooled.

At least my mom didn't pack raw fish for lunch. I had a bagel with cream cheese and chocolate milk. That was the highlight of my day, Diary.

With love from a fourth grader who will always have three brothers,
Jessica Allman

August 29
6:50 in the morning

Dear Diary,

I woke up before my alarm today because the bats have invaded my stomach once again. I thought I'd write a quick note to you to help calm me down. Diary, what do I do about the Olivia Michaels of the world? I can't be eating ice pops in the nurse's office every day!

Okay. Here's a plan. I'll get revenge. I'll look at her "All About Me" poster and tell her it's boring. Nah! Just imagining that conversation makes me feel like a worm. Okay, I need a better plan. IGNORE! I'll ignore her! Today, according to my attendance book, Olivia Michaels will be absent from Mrs. Lindner's class. Hear no evil. See no evil. Feel no evil.

I'll let you know how that works out, Diary. Wish me luck. Ben just woke up so I guess I'd better start getting ready for school. I feel a little calmer, Diary, but this entry is still. . .

From a very nervous fourth grader,
Jessica

August 29
7:30 at night

Dear D,

Well, I made it through the day thanks to the Lindsay Beth Silbers of the world. And you know what, Diary? It was actually an okay day. It all started when I was walking to Mrs. Lindner's classroom with Lindsay and she told me that Olivia started to cry yesterday after Mrs. Lindner took me to the nurse's office. It seems as though Olivia Michaels has a heart after all, and it was hurting after those unkind words came flying out of her mouth. At least that's what she told Lindsay. So Lindsay suggested to her that she write me a note to apologize, and Lindsay warned me that I would find this note on my desk when I walked in this morning. As usual, Lindsay was right, except the note was on my chair, not my desk. It was in a pink envelope covered with hearts and I pretended to be surprised to see it there because I could feel Olivia's eyes watching me as I sat down to read it. Here's what it said, Diary:

Dear Jessica:

I'm not sure how to say this but I said something really mean to you yesterday about your family and I shouldn't have said it, and I'm sorry if I hurt your feelings. I'm sorry about what happened to your brother.

I hope we can be friends.

From,
Olivia

I wrote back to her and told her not to worry about what she'd said yesterday, and I told her that her note made me feel much better. I wasn't about to say anything more than that, though. I'm not exactly eager to be her friend, so I just didn't say anything about that part yet. I think she really does want to be my friend, though, because she sat next to me and Lindsay at lunch and shared her Oreos with us. I guess she's not so bad after all. And I guess kids don't think I'm as much of a weirdo as I thought they might. We had to choose partners for gym today and two girls, Carly and Alicia, asked at the same time to be my partner. We all giggled and then asked our gym teacher if we could triple up and she said it would be fine. We had to make up a dance and we made up a really cool one. Wish I could show it to you, Diary, but I can't do it very well without my partners.

I'm feeling pretty tired. Remember I wrote to you really early this morning? Time to snooze. Thanks for being with me morning and night.

Your friend,
Jessica

Dear Diary,

My mom had the bright idea to schedule a visit with Faye after school today because I think she realizes that Ben and I are feeling quite topsy-turvy. All this back to school stuff is pretty nerve-wracking. When Faye asked us how things were going, the room filled with quiet. The quiet didn't last too long, though, because Ricky burst in with milk bubbles and cookie crumbs on his lips eager to tell Faye about the frog he'd caught for mom. He was even more excited to tell her he would soon be swimming better than the frog because his swim lessons were making him "very smart about swimming."

After clapping for Ricky, Faye looked at Ben and me. I was just getting ready to share my story about Olivia when Ben suddenly announced that he really appreciated the "Sorry" cards his classmates made for him in school today. Are you surprised, Diary? I sure was! It turns out that at recess kids were asking Ben questions about what happened to Matt, and after explaining for the third time Ben got tired of answering them. When he got back to class, he asked Mr. Douglas if he could explain to the whole class that Matt passed away.

Diary, they say brothers and sisters can be nothing alike, and in this case I have to agree. I never could have stood up and spoken to my whole class about Matt. I know I don't have to hide it like a "bad secret" but I just want to be with kids in a normal way. No announcements about my private life, just normal talking and stuff. I guess Ben is different that way. He likes to set things straight, just like he did with Joey Gilman. He's able to be really honest and I think that's a lucky way to be.

Well, there was an uncomfortable quiet in Ben's class after he finished explaining Matt's story. Mr. Douglas broke the silence by asking each student to write a card to Ben. One note from Olivia Michaels was enough for me, Diary, but Ben felt really good about receiving twenty-two! Faye thought it was very special to have those notes and she was really proud of Ben for being so brave. I think having that collection of cards makes Ben feel more a part of his class, like kids can really know him now. He's smart, that Ben. Fourth graders can definitely learn something from second graders.

Diary, I want to tell you what Faye said about the Olivia Michaels situation, but I can barely keep my eyes open. I promise I'll give you all the details tomorrow.

Love ya,
Jessica

August 31
7:38 at night

Dear Diary,

School felt a little easier today because I reminded myself every now and then about my conversation with Faye yesterday, which I was too tired to write about last night but I really want to share with you now. Diary, she told me she was really proud of me, too, because I handled my problem in "Jessica's way." I prefer to keep things private and I'm entitled to my privacy. She totally understood why I made a bee-line for the nurse's office. Privacy! She explained that it was hard for each of us to go back to school because we were partly a different Jessica and Ben than we used to be and we needed to get used to this new part of ourselves in our own way. If that meant sharing feelings with the whole class, great! If that meant sharing feelings only with our closest friends and family, that was fine, too. What matters most, according to Faye, is that we go to school each day (so much for my homeschooling theory!), because school helps every part of our self—old and new—grow. She promises that most days will feel a little easier than the day before and I have a feeling she's right.

And of course—she reminded us—Matt loved school and he would want us to be happy there. That point gives me courage, Diary.

So that kind of explains why school was a little easier today. Plus, I'm having fun working on my dance with Carly and Alicia. Plus, Mrs. Lindner gave us extra time to play outside because it was a beautiful day, and I saw four different butterflies (that I secretly named Matt, Jessie, Ben and Ricky). Double plus: Mrs. Lindner assigned our permanent seats today. I'm neighbors with Lindsay Beth Silber, and my dance partner, Carly, while both William Kingsley and Olivia Michaels are miles away from my desk. A purrfect arrangement . . . although I have to admit that William and Olivia are acting pretty normal toward me unlike that dreadful Tuesday.

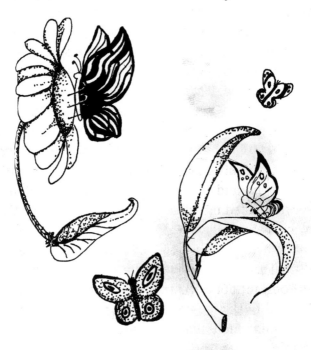

From a slightly less nervous fourth grader,
Jessica

September 1
7:15 at night

Diary, Diary, Diary!

I came upstairs earlier than usual tonight because I have so much to share with you. It's good news but the kind that's so powerful it makes it hard to catch your breath. First let me report that I was elected to be our class representative for the student government. That's a shocker, Diary, because everyone in our class had to vote and I was the one the kids chose! Jessica Allman, imagine that! I have to say I made a pretty good speech before the vote saying how I would do some fundraising to purchase a class pet—a frog, of course. Also, I would set up a food drive at Thanksgiving time and make baskets for families that don't have enough food (the Allmans certainly have a large basket collection to share!) And I would ask for more balls, jump ropes and sidewalk chalk for recess. I guess everyone liked my ideas because—my first student government meeting is tomorrow!

Ok, so I came home from school today feeling pretty happy that I never talked my parents into the homeschool option, and after some cheese and crackers I went upstairs to do my first homework assignment. I felt like things were going so well, and I felt proud and brave, Diary. I closed my eyes shut in a moment of joy and suddenly pictured Matt giving me a big hug. And then I did it, Diary. I needed a pencil and paper for my math problems so I walked straight into Ben's room, bee-line to Matt's desk. I opened the top drawer and felt my heart thump hard in my chest (at least it didn't stop beating). My eyes sort of froze on the collection of his stuff in the drawer . . . his student government membership card, his address book, a N.Y. Knicks keychain, a math award. I looked at all of it and thought . . . . here's a glimpse of Matt's world, untouched, unchanged . . . it's almost like a rewind button, backspace to the real Allman family. I didn't want to move a thing.

Then I couldn't stop myself. I opened every drawer and touched, smelled and studied whatever I could find. A pencil case filled with M&M's!!!! (Now I know where the M&M's came from on Lindsay's sleepover date!) His autographed pictures of athletes, old school reports, his baseball cards, an "All About Me Book" that he made in nursery school. There's a page in it with a drawing of Mom and Dad bringing me home from the hospital. I know it's me because the teacher labeled the page "Welcome home baby sister Jessica."

I was shuffling through his school supplies drawer, which I discovered to be the bottom drawer, when I saw a little red notebook labeled M.A.'s New Year's Resolutions 1998. Seeing this made my eyes go blurry and they started to sting. I wondered if my privacy code should take effect at this moment. Hadn't I looked through enough of Matt's stuff? I had looked through plenty, but this little red book of hopes and promises pulled me hardest of all. I just had to peek inside. Whether or not I should've done it . . . I did it . . . and Diary, I'm glad I did. I felt so proud of Matt. He had a heart brimming with goodness and a desire to be the best person he could be. This notebook is an absolute gift I will have forever. I'm going to devote your next blank page to his resolutions, Diary. Be prepared! You know how most people set one or two goals for a new year? Matt made 20! I think you'll know what I mean when I say it's the kind of powerful information that makes it hard to catch your breath.

Matt Allman's New Year's Resolutions 1998

1. I shall not lie to my friends or family. I will be honest and trustworthy.
2. I shall not steal books or papers and take responsibility for my actions.
3. I shall not curse or swear in emotion or freely.
4. I will not take my parents for granted and I will not beg for clothes or anything that I need or do not need.
5. I will use my own mind and I will not do anything I think is wrong.
6. I will not push my brothers and sister around.
7. I will not do anything behind Mom's or Dad's back that they would be displeased about.
8. I will not misbehave in religious school and I will show respect for my religion.
9. I will try harder in basketball and show people why I am the captain of the Davis Dolphins.

10. I will cut down on TV and pay more attention to books.
11. I shall not lose my temper in times of anger.
12. I shall not take my allowance for granted and I will fully complete my chores.
13. I will show more respect for my music teacher.
14. I will not make a mess at the dinner table with my food.
15. I will not dump my food under the table even if I do not like it.
16. I will take better care of my teeth.
17. I will not instigate Ricky and make him hit me and fight me.
18. At camp, I will write more letters.
19. I will try to learn new things and explore unexplored territory.
20. I will be more attuned toward my family.

Diary, I still feel that big hug coming from Matt. I don't know how the courage burst out of me to look through his desk, but I would guess it has a lot to do with a part of Matt being inside me forever. I don't think he would mind that I looked. I would explain to him that such important thoughts need to be shared with the world or at least with his family! I really respect all of his intentions to become the best person possible. I hope I can take over this wish for him. I'm glad I'm going to school because I know it's the right way to grow into the best person I can be.

I really need to find Ben and Ricky. It's definitely time for another kids' meeting. Matt may not be here to fulfill these resolutions but the rest of the Allman kids could certainly take on the challenge. It's unexplored territory all right, but our oldest brother has shown us the way.

Signing off for now.

The second oldest Allman kid,
Jessie

About the Author

Jodi Scheinfeld began her career as a publicist with Arbor House Books in New York City. She soon switched to teaching after studying for and receiving a Masters Degree in English and Comparative Literature at Columbia University. She taught High School English for seven years until her second child was born, and has been a stay at home mom for the last twenty years, raising her children. During this time, she has done some freelance magazine writing, along with extensive volunteer work in her community and local public schools.

In 1998 after her oldest son, Jeremy, died at ten years of age, Jodi and her husband Rob established the Jeremy Scheinfeld Foundation for Kids to benefit children of all ages. It remains very important to both of them to engage in pursuits that honor their son's memory. The foundation supports programs and projects including, research, arts, scholarship and athletics—all for children. Jodi is gratified to publish her first novel, *A Sister's Diary*, to help children understand loss and empower them with the knowledge that there are ways to support themselves through it and build a hopeful and beautiful future that is always connected to their loved ones. Proceeds from this book will go to Jeremy's Foundation.

Jodi and Rob are also camp safety advocates, have a website to raise awareness about camp safety (campsafetyguide.com), and speak publicly about the importance of camp safety. They were successful in the state of New York in improving camp safety legislation, and were able to partner nationally with the American Camp Association to develop a staff training DVD entitled "Who Will Care When I'm Not There?" used today by hundreds of camps across the country.

Jodi resides in the state of New York with Rob and their five children, all of whom are the light and loves of her life. Her hobbies include ballet, knitting, gardening and, of course, reading.